GETTING THE MOST OUT OF YOUR VITAMINS AND MINERALS

It's one thing to understand the fundamentals of nutrition, and it's quite another to know how to make vitamins and minerals work for you. Over the last several years, literally thousands of articles on the preventive and therapeutic uses of vitamins and minerals have been published in medical journals once hostile toward the use of nutritional supplements. Medicine now recognizes that vitamins and minerals can ease the symptoms of common ailments, such as colds and sore throats, and effectively prevent and treat such life-threatening diseases as cancer and heart disease. For consumers, this book provides the latest information on what the leading vitamins and minerals do—and how to make the most of them. And for health care professionals, this book's complete references make it easy to find the medical journal articles where this information originally appeared.

GETTING THE MOST OUT OF YOUR VITAMINS AND MINERALS

THE LATEST EVIDENCE ON HOW THEY FIGHT DISEASE AND HELP YOU LIVE LONGER AND BETTER

by Jack Challem

With detailed citations for physicians and other health professionals.

KeatsPublishing, Inc. 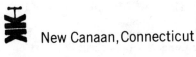 New Canaan, Connecticut

Getting the Most Out of Your Vitamins and Minerals is not intended as medical advice. Its intent is solely informational and educational. Please consult a health professional should the need for one be indicated.

Some phrases, passages and quotes have previously appeared in *Bestways, Health News & Review, EastWest, Natural Health, LET'S LIVE*, and the *Journal of Orthomolecular Medicine*.

Good Health Guides are published by
Keats Publishing, Inc.
27 Pine Street (Box 876)
New Canaan, Connecticut 06840-0876

CONTENTS

VITAMIN THERAPY COMES OF AGE

It's the 1990s—and vitamin therapy has come of age.

The question is not whether you should take vitamin and mineral supplements. It's how you can make the most of them to improve your health and live a longer, fuller life.

Twenty years ago, people who took vitamin and mineral supplements were often considered eccentric, if not downright wacky. And most doctors knew as much about vitamins as they did about astrophysics. That was unfortunate, because vitamins have always been a lot easier to understand and use.

Today, if you scan the *New York Times, Newsweek,* or *Time* magazine, you're more likely than ever to find articles extolling the health benefits of vitamins and minerals. And if you visit a medical library, you'll discover even bigger surprises. Open the pages of leading medical journals—such as *The Journal of the American Medical Association, The New England Journal of Medicine, Diabetes, Lancet,* and *The American Journal of Cardiology*—and you'll find solid scientific evidence supporting the benefits of vitamins and minerals: vitamins C and E for preventing heart disease and cancer, calcium for lowering blood pressure, magnesium for controlling cardiac arrhythmias, chromium for helping diabetes, zinc for fighting sore throats and colds, and lots more.

Thousands of articles on the therapeutic benefits of vitamins and minerals are now published annually in medical journals. And they are more easily accessible to doctors, medical reporters, and the average person. By typing a few keystrokes on a computer terminal at any medical school library, people can scan Medline and other computer databases and, for example, instantly retrieve summaries of the 600 articles published on vitamin E in the last year alone.

Thanks to this surge of research, we're learning volumes about how nutrients maintain and restore health. And as a consequence, increasing numbers of physicians are incorporating nutritional therapies into their medical practices. Dieticians or doctors who still argue that vitamins and minerals have no value simply aren't keeping up with the latest research.

What accounts for the growing acceptance of vitamin therapy? A number of factors. First, in the early 1970s, spurred by Nobel laureate Linus Pauling's book, *Vitamin C and the Common Cold,* researchers around the world began studying vitamins and minerals with greater intensity than in the past.

Second, unlike their predecessors in the 1940s and 1950s, these researchers have had the sophisticated tools of molecular biology to unravel the precise details of how and why vitamins and minerals work. While the average person isn't interested in such minutiae, they are important to the "medical establishment" that has incredible sway on how doctors practice medicine.

Third, the growing acceptance of the "free-radical" theory of aging and disease has opened the door to vitamins and minerals, many of which naturally control these harmful substances.

Fourth, vitamin and mineral therapy is increasingly recognized as an extraordinarily safe and low-cost method of preventing and treating disease, which has the potential to reduce our nation's immense health-care costs.

Perhaps not too surprisingly, today's researchers have largely confirmed most of the claims for vitamins and minerals made over the last 50 years. And they're discovering even newer benefits from taking supplements.

To keep pace with these advances, this Good Health Guide's objective is to help you make the most of your vitamins and minerals. Instead of repeating the well-known but basic information on the nutritional roles of vitamins and minerals, *this guide focuses on the latest research and clinical findings related to their therapeutic uses.* While this book isn't intended to be the most comprehensive discussion of vitamin therapy, it is designed as a guide to the vitamins and minerals you're most likely to benefit from.

It's best, of course, to work with your physician in employing vitamin therapy. Share this book with him or her. If he's still skeptical, draw his attention to the original medical journal references at the back of this book. Your doctor can easily obtain the original medical articles through the nearest medical school library. Encourage him to do so.

WHY YOU SHOULD TAKE VITAMIN AND MINERAL SUPPLEMENTS

Reason #1: Odds are you don't get enough vitamins and minerals from your diet. And those that you do get probably aren't used all that efficiently.

We've all known people who seem healthy regardless of how they abuse their bodies—and those who do everything right but still have difficulty achieving real health. The late Roger Williams, Ph.D., discoverer of the B vitamin pantothenic acid, explained why in his brilliant concept of biochemical individuality: Just as we look different on the outside, the internal workings of our bodies—and the way we use nutrients—differ greatly.[1]

Williams' theory of biochemical individuality explains that everyone needs the same 50-odd nutrients, but they need these nutrients in dramatically different amounts. In his classic *Nutrition Against Disease*, Williams wrote that "every individual has nutritional needs which differ *quantitatively*, with respect to each separate nutrient, from his neighbors. . . . Each individual has a pattern of needs all his own." These nutritional needs may vary by dozens, even hundreds, of times.[2]

Williams elaborated in a 1976 article: "It is easy to see differences on the outside of the human body. People come in all sizes and shapes—tall or short, fat or lean, bald or bushy-haired, large ears or petite, snub noses or Jimmy Durante specials, blue eyes or brown. . . . Less well known, but even more startling is the differentiation of our internal organs. Autopsies have shown that stomachs, hearts, colons, livers, intestines, nasal passages, and muscles all exhibit wide variations in size and shape—producing individualized anatomical, physiological, biochemical, neurological, endocrinological and probably even psychological problems."[3]

In an interview in 1977, Williams explained that biochemical individuality "simply tells us that body chemistries are not the same. Two people of about the same height and weight have about the same total metabolism, but the *details* of chemical reactions taking place in their bodies may be very different. Certain reactions will take place ten times as fast in one individual as another. This makes our nutritional needs different and has a lot of other effects."[4]

Williams' concept of biochemical individuality also means that the federal government's widely promoted recommended dietary allowances (RDAs) have limited value. The RDAs, he said, "apply to only a hypothetical average person which doesn't exist. The typical person probably has some needs which are very far from average."[5]

The RDAs ignore the wide variations in human biochemistry and, as a blanket statement of nutritional needs, may do more harm than good. Jeffrey Blumberg, Ph.D., professor of nutrition at Tufts University, recently said that "the U.S. RDA is based on the prevention of deficiency diseases and is targeted to normal growth and maintenance of apparently healthy people. They [the RDA committee] never said they were anything else. The RDAs are increasingly irrelevant to today's public health concerns, and reducing the risk of heart disease, cancer, cataracts, arthritis, and other diseases is not a criteria for the RDAs."[6]

Reason #2: You can use vitamin and mineral supplements to "vaccinate" yourself against an unnatural environment.

Most of us live in an environment that is, to one degree or another, unnatural and contaminated. Our bodies must endure air and water pollution, increased ultraviolet rays from sunlight, ionizing radiation from nuclear energy sources, nonionizing radiation from radio and microwaves, pesticides and an assortment of chemicals added to foods, cigarette smoke, carbon monoxide in auto exhaust, formaldehyde released from new carpeting and building materials, and, last but not least, increasingly virulent infections.

The biochemical fulcrum for all of these assaults on our bodies is increased formation of free radicals, molecular fragments that age our cells faster and make us more susceptible to cancer, heart disease, and other diseases. Although free-radical formation can be slowed with antioxidants, we face a quandary: Just when we need these antioxidants more than ever before, our diets suffer from an unprecedented decline in them. The nutritional value of our food supply has diminished from overworked farmlands, poor or improper soil fertilization, and from progressive nutrient losses during shipping, partitioning, processing, cooking and reheating. If the antioxidants in our diet have historically constituted a major defense, then this defense has been seriously weakened.

To compensate for some of these losses and to bolster our biological defenses, vitamin and mineral supplements can serve as "heroic countermeasures against an unnatural environment," contends Emanuel Cheraskin, M.D., D.M.D., professor emeritus of the University of Alabama.

"We are pretty much a function of nurture and nature," he said in an interview. "What we got from our parents, we can't do a lot about. What we get in our environment—the air we breathe, the water we drink—we can do a little but not a lot about. The food we eat is the most controllable element in our environment.

"The question is 'What can we do to vaccinate ourselves?' " he continued. "For every cigarette you smoke, for example, you need more vitamin C. The RDA for vitamin C is 60 mg. For smokers, it's officially 100 mg—but that's crazy. Smokers need far more. You also need more vitamin C if you take laxatives, antibiotics, or the contraceptive pill. The answer is that you can vaccinate yourself with vitamins."[7]

Cheraskin added that as our environment becomes more chemically complex, we suffer from more degenerative diseases. "Vitamins and minerals are part of the answer to these problems. In a situation where we're blasted by so much, we need electron donors like vitamin C to compensate for the tremendous amount of damage."

Reason #3: If "free radicals" cause disease, then "antioxidant" vitamins and minerals are the logical—and natural—way to protect yourself.

Scientists have known about free radicals for decades, but only over the past ten years have advances in molecular biology pointed unequivocally to their role in virtually every disease and disorder. Free radicals are molecular fragments that damage normal molecules by stripping away electrons, resulting in oxidation and reducing the efficiency of cells. Unless neutralized, free radicals become a biochemical snowball—progressively stripping away still more electrons from healthy molecules and cells.

So what, you say? When free radicals are not stopped, a cell's deoxyribonucleic acid (DNA) is altered and it cannot precisely replicate itself. The replicated cell is different—less efficient, with metabolic aberrations, and with a reduced life span. It's known as aging. Multiply it by several billion times and you start to look and feel old before your time.

In one view of the process, Douglas C. Wallace, Ph.D., chairman of the department of genetics and molecular medicine at the Emory University School of Medicine in Atlanta, explained that aging begins when too many mutations occur within a cell's mitochondrial DNA (mtDNA), interfering with energy production.

This energy-producing process, called oxidative phosphorylation (OXPHOS) is influenced by genetics, environmental poisons, and nutrient intake. Writing in the May 1, 1992 *Science*, Wallace explained that "the OXPHOS system declines with age. . . . One possible cause of this age-related decline in OXPHOS as well as the high mtDNA mutation rate is damage of mtDNA by oxygen free radicals."[8]

Disease symptoms, he pointed out, appear when the target organ reaches an oxidative point of no return. "The most likely mechanism is the accumulation of damage to mtDNA by oxidation. . . ." Even worse, the mutated mtDNA replicates faster than normal mtDNA, accelerating the aging process.

In conclusion, Wallace said that preventive therapy with antioxidants "may ultimately allow individuals at risk for a variety of degenerative diseases to avoid developing symptoms." Such a view underpins the justification and growing acceptance of vitamin therapy. As it turns out, the most powerful antioxidants are natural ones: vitamins C and E, selenium, glutathione, and coenzyme Q10. These nutrients serve as electron donors, replacing the electrons taken by free radicals and minimizing their molecular and cellular damage.

Reason #4: Vitamin and mineral supplements can help you achieve optimal health.

In 1968, Linus Pauling coined the phrase "orthomolecular medicine" to describe a relatively natural means of straightening out the cells of the body. Pauling stressed the benefits of achieving "optimal molecular concentrations of substances normally present in the body . . . vitamins, essential amino acids, essential fatty acids." He argued that these optimal amounts were higher than the "minimum" or "recommended" daily amounts generally promoted by the government and dieticians for health.[9]

The RDAs, he explained in an interview, are fine as a baseline for a person's bottom-line nutritional needs but not as a standard for optimal nutrition. "The RDAs are the amounts of vitamins and minerals that prevent nearly all persons from developing signs of corresponding nutritional deficiencies. But how much should a person take to be in the best of health, not just ordinary poor health? These amounts are in excess of the RDAs, especially vitamin C, the optimal doses of which may be 200 times the RDA." Pauling went on to explain that, at age 91, he was taking 300 times the RDA of vitamin C, 80 times the RDA of vitamin E, and 20 times the RDA of the B-complex vitamins.[10]

Pauling believes that vitamin supplements are a technological advance capable of ushering in a new era of optimal health. They can prime the body's cells to perform at their genetic peak of efficiency, slowing the aging process and minimizing degenerative diseases.

While that may be true of all vitamins and minerals, vitamin C may be fundamentally different from—and far more important than—the others. Pauling cites the seminal research of the late Irwin Stone, a biochemist who explained that virtually every plant and animal species produces vitamin C ($C_6H_8O_6$) from chemically similar glucose ($C_6H_{12}O_6$). Humans lack a single enzyme, L-gulonolactone oxidase, needed to accomplish this conversion, as do some higher primates and a handful of other animals. Our evolutionary ancestors may have lost this enzyme, says Pauling, as a result of an evolutionary accident. For some reason, the primates (Anthropoidea suborder) successfully evolved without needing the metabolic machinery to produce vitamin C.[11,12]

In his classic book, *The Healing Factor: Vitamin C Against Disease*, Stone observed that, across the animal kingdom, the daily nonstressed rate of vitamin C production hovers around 85 mg per pound of body weight. He used the goat as a model comparable in weight, diet, and physiology to a human adult. The liver of a 150-pound goat, he explained, manufactures about 13,000 mg of vitamin C during a typical, nonstressful day. When under stress, such as during an infection, the goat's production of vitamin C increases as much as three times.

In this view, high doses of vitamin C supplements may not be so much a dietary substance as a matter of replenishing "a product of man's original metabolism" to correct an "inherited enzyme disease." If true, supplemental vitamin C, in high doses, may be absolutely necessary for attaining optimal health.[13]

GETTING THE MOST OUT OF YOUR VITAMINS

BETA-CAROTENE

Beta-carotene reverses the immune system depression typical of AIDS and chronic fatigue syndrome. In addition, beta- and alpha-carotene prevent, and may even cure, some types of cancer.

Beta-Carotene Fights AIDS and Chronic Fatigue

According to the latest evidence, high doses of beta-carotene can fight some of the most debilitating and deadly diseases of the 1990s: acquired immune deficiency syndrome (AIDS), chronic fatigue syndrome (CFS), and cancer.

In February 1993, Gregg Coodley, M.D., of the Oregon Health Sciences University in Portland, announced his findings that beta-carotene supplements increased the number of disease-fighting immune cells produced by the body. He had confirmed earlier research by Harinder Garewal, M.D., of the University of Arizona Cancer Center, Tucson, showing that high doses of beta-carotene could strengthen the immune systems of people infected with the human immunodeficiency virus (HIV), which causes AIDS.[14]

Coodley's study of 21 patients infected with HIV found that taking 180 mg of supplemental beta-carotene daily increased the number of protective white blood cells—called CD4, T4, or T-helper cells—by an average of 13 percent. Twenty of the patients were also receiving the AIDS drug AZT, but the benefits from the beta-carotene appeared to be independent of those from the AZT.[15]

A CD4 count in healthy people is about 1,000 per deciliter of blood, and the diagnosis of AIDS is made when the CD4 count is 200 or less. When the study began, the patients' CD4 counts ranged from zero to 700. By increasing the CD4 count, Coodley slowed the progression from HIV to AIDS, extending the lifespan of the infected people.

The 180 mg dose of beta-carotene is equivalent to 300,000 IU of vitamin A activity, but there are no toxic effects from beta-carotene over-dose. Coodley acknowledged he wasn't sure why the beta-carotene helped. He speculated that it might be because the nutrient increased production of the CD4 cells or prevented their destruction.

In an interview, Coodley said he wasn't sure whether beta-carotene would have an effect on other infections, such as colds and flus. However, he thinks that the nutrient "may have benefits with other conditions that result in a suppressed immune system, such as chronic fatigue syndrome."[16]

Indeed, there are many parallels between AIDS and CFS. Both diseases are relatively new and both suppress immune defenses. In addition, both AIDS and CFS patients tend to suffer from yeast infections, dementia, unusual forms of cancer, and antibody responses to diseases they have never been exposed to.

Recognizing that many people will take beta-carotene supplements on their own, without a physician's guidance, Coodley added, "It's a substance that's hard to do yourself a lot of harm with. We don't have proof that this will work on a sustained period, but I am hoping to do a follow-up study to determine what happens. The effect may be more significant for people with a more depressed immune system."

Beta- and Alpha-Carotene Fight Cancer

In their inimitable way of making nutrients sound like drugs, conventional physicians commonly refer to beta-carotene supplements as a form of "chemo-prevention." Perhaps a more appropriate term would be "nutri-prevention." The body converts beta-carotene, found abundantly in green and yellow vegetables, to vitamin A. Although vitamin A has anti-cancer properties, the latest evidence indicates that many of beta-carotene's benefits are independent of the vitamin.

To date, more than 70 studies have shown that beta-carotene decreases a person's risk of developing cancer, and Harinder Garewal, M.D., has been one of the leading researchers. In one study, he demonstrated that even very low doses of beta-carotene can reverse precancerous lesions called leukoplakia. The condition, most common in people who smoke tobacco and drink alcohol, is characterized by white patches on the inside of the mouth and throat. Of greater concern, leukoplakia is often a prelude to head and neck cancers, which include tumors of the mouth, tongue, lips, pharynx and larynx.

Dr. Garewal treated 25 patients with leukoplakia by giving them a 30-mg capsule of beta-carotene daily, equivalent to the beta-carotene in six carrots (or to 50,000 IU of vitamin A activity), for six months. In 17 of the patients—roughly three-quarters—the leukoplakias shrank by at least 50 percent. In several of the patients, the leukoplakias completely disappeared. However, the condition returned when patients stopped taking the beta-carotene supplement.[17,18]

According to an article in the *Berkeley Wellness Letter*, published by the University of California, most people don't eat anything close to the amount of beta-carotene needed for health.[19] One survey, reported the newsletter, showed that 49 percent of Americans eat only one vegetable a day and 41 percent eat no fruit whatsoever.

Although beta-carotene appears to be the most biologically active carotene in people, it is actually only one of hundreds. According to a report in the National Cancer Institute's *Cancer Weekly*, a team of Japanese researchers headed by Michiaki Murakoshi, Ph.D., discovered that *alpha*-carotene was ten times more effective than beta-carotene in fighting cancer.[20] This lesser known alpha-carotene accounts for about one-third of the carotene found in carrots and about 5 percent of the carotene found in most beta-carotene supplements.

In one study, Murakoshi and his colleagues at the Kyota Prefectural University in Japan found that alpha-carotene suppressed the growth of several types of malignant tumors, including neuroblastomas, pancreatic cancer, glioblastoma, and gastric cancer. In a follow-up study, Murakoshi discovered that alpha-carotene was ten times more effective than beta-carotene in suppressing the growth of neuroblastoma cancer cells. In fact, the suppression of cancer cells began less than 18 hours after the administration of alpha-carotene.

THE B-COMPLEX VITAMINS

Several of the B vitamins prevent heart disease, while others are helpful in carpal tunnel syndrome and multiple sclerosis.

B6, Folic Acid, and Choline Prevent Heart Disease

While elevated cholesterol and triglyceride levels are among the most recognizable risk factors for heart disease, another heart hazard has emerged from the shadows: *homocysteine*. Once thought to be only a sign of a rare congenital disorder, high levels of homocysteine are now recognized as an independent risk factor in heart disease.

Homocysteine is known to be atherogenic—that is, it attacks heart tissue. While not a nutrient, it is a biochemical produced during the breakdown of methionine, an essential amino acid. However, as long as the diet contains ample vitamin B6, folic acid, and choline, homocysteine exists only briefly before being converted to cystathionine, which is harmless.

To demonstrate the significance of homocysteine, Meir Stampfer, M.D., and colleagues at the Brigham and Women's Hospital and Harvard Medical School, Boston, analyzed the blood samples of 14,916 male physicians. Although none of the doctors had suffered a heart attack when the study began, 271 did during the next five years.

Stampfer discovered that 31 of the doctors suffering heart attacks had extremely high blood levels of homocysteine, which did not correspond to any other risk factors, such as smoking or cholesterol. "However, we found significant inverse correlations between homocyst[e]ine levels and intake of several vitamins," he wrote in *The Journal of the American Medical Association.*[21]

Most striking, the doctors with the highest homocysteine levels— above the 95th percentile—were three times more likely to suffer from a heart attack than doctors with homocysteine levels below the 90th percentile.

Stampfer pointed out that high levels of vitamin intake are typically associated with low levels of homocysteine. Ironically, he observed, the physicians in the study were likely to eat better than the average person. In other words, most people may be in far worse shape.

For example, a dietary study published in the *American Journal of Clinical Nutrition* found that one-third of elderly, low-income people were deficient in B6, because of poor diets or because they smoked tobacco.[22] Another study, reported in the *American Journal of Clinical Nutrition,* found that half of all Americans do not obtain adequate folic acid (folate) from their diets.[23]

In light of this, Stampfer noted the ease of vitamin therapy. "Nutritional surveys suggest that suboptimal intake of vitamin B6 and folate are not uncommon in the United States. . . . Elevated homocyst[e]ine levels can often be normalized by modest doses of folate (1 to 5 mg/day). For cases that are resistant to this therapy, the addition of vitamin B6, choline, or betaine is often effective.

These supplements at the recommended dosages have few or no side effects under most circumstances."

Although this was the latest study pointing to homocysteine as a risk factor in heart disease, similar research has been conducted for more than 30 years, beginning with Kilmer McCully, M.D., of Harvard. Over the past several years, research on homocysteine has accelerated.

For example, physicians Robert Clarke and Ian Graham of the Department of Cardiology, Adelaide Hospital, Dublin, reported that almost one-third of patients with coronary artery disease or peripheral artery disease had high homocysteine levels. In contrast, homocysteine levels were normal in patients without heart disease, according to an article they wrote for the *New England Journal of Medicine*.[24]

Similarly, Bo Israelsson, M.D., of Malmö General Hospital in Sweden, found that five patients who survived their first heart attack at a relatively early age (under 55) had abnormally high blood levels of homocysteine and low levels of folate and B12. Israelsson wrote in the journal *Atherosclerosis* that "moderate homocysteinemia exists in a high proportion of men with low conventional risk factors for arteriosclerotic disease . . . if moderately increased plasma homocysteine can be verified as a risk factor for arteriosclerotic disease, simple and safe therapy is available. We have previously found and recently confirmed that all levels, not only high levels, of total plasma homocysteine can be reduced simply by giving a supplement of . . . folic acid a day."[25]

According to homocysteine expert Manuel René Malinow, M.D., of the Oregon Regional Primate Research Center in Beaverton, up to 15 percent of people with coronary artery disease may have high homocysteine levels. Among those who have had a stroke, the percentage is 40 percent. And among those with intermittent claudication ("restless legs"), 35 percent have elevated homocysteine levels. Meanwhile, among otherwise healthy people, only about 5 percent of the people have high homocysteine levels in their blood.

B6 and B2 Relieve Carpal Tunnel Syndrome

Many people believe that the widespread use of personal computers is responsible for the alarming incidence of carpal tunnel syndrome. The condition is characterized by pain and numbness in the hand caused by pressure in the carpal tunnel of the wrist.

The symptomatic similarities to arthritis were evident to John Ellis,

M.D., of Mt. Pleasant, Texas, who has found the B-complex vitamins excellent therapeutic agents. He explored the treatment of carpal tunnel syndrome with Karl Folkers, Ph.D., director of the Institute for Biomedical Research at the University of Texas, Austin.

After first conducting an unsuccessful double-blind study with B6 for six weeks, they decided to duplicate the study for 12 weeks. Over this longer period, symptoms of carpal tunnel syndrome decreased as B6 activity increased, according to their article in the *Annals of the New York Academy of Sciences.*[26]

One particular case, a 40-year-old male with crippled hands, illustrated the benefits of B6. He was given 2 mg of B6—the recommended daily allowance—for two months. Ellis and Folkers measured slight increases in an enzyme associated with B6 activity. The patient still had symptoms but did show "slight clinical improvement." When his dose was increased to 100 mg, enzymes indicative of B6 activity increased substantially and, in another two months, his symptoms completely disappeared.

The patient was then given an identical-looking placebo, but was not told of the change. "The patient strongly complained that pyridoxine was no longer effective . . . his symptoms returned on placebo. The need for adequate daily vitamin B6 was evident." When the patient was again given 100 mg of B6 daily, his condition improved.

Ellis and Folkers then described the treatment of "a typical patient with the carpal tunnel syndrome first with riboflavin (B2) and then with combined riboflavin and pyridoxine (B6) . . . the results were that riboflavin therapy alone was effective biochemically, subjectively, and objectively . . . treatment with combined riboflavin and pyridoxine was even more effective than when riboflavin alone was administered. Therefore, the carpal tunnel syndrome is the clinical result of deficiencies of both. . . ."

B12 May Help Multiple Sclerosis

Thumb through all the medical textbooks you can find, but you still won't find multiple sclerosis (MS) listed as a complication of vitamin B12 deficiency. So there was considerable medical interest when E. H. Reynolds, M.D., of the Department of Neurology, Kings College Hospital, London, described ten MS patients (seven women and three men) with B12 deficiency in the *Archives of Neurology.* Perhaps even more noteworthy, eight of the patients were under age 40, an unusual age for B12 deficiency.[27]

"In a period of five years, we observed three cases of multiple sclerosis associated with unusual vitamin B12 deficiencies," explained Reynolds. "Following presentation of these patients to the Association of British Neurologists, seven additional cases have been referred by other neurologists in a one-year period."

Reynolds speculated that there might be a relationship between pernicious anemia and MS in some patients. "It is theoretically possible that vitamin B12 deficiency, whatever its cause, could render the patient more vulnerable to the putative viral and/or immunological mechanisms widely suspected in multiple sclerosis." Even more perplexing, tests showed no evidence of peripheral neuropathy, the most common sign of B12 deficiency.

The obvious question, of course, is whether treatment with vitamin B12 offers clinical improvement for MS patients. Only two of Reynolds' patients have been followed for more than a year while receiving B12, and these patients' conditions have not deteriorated.

"It is relevant that for some 30 years, there has been a tendency to treat multiple sclerosis with injections of vitamin B12," added Reynolds. "Although this is done for placebo purposes, this was not the original intention, and some patients are impressed with their neurologic benefit . . . The ten patients described herein suggest that interest in the subject should be reawakened."

In a follow-up study of 29 consecutive MS patients, Reynolds discovered that all of them were severely deficient in B12, making the association more than a simple medical curiosity. "There is a significant association between MS and disturbed B12 metabolism. Vitamin B12 deficiency should always be looked for in patients with MS," he wrote in *Archives of Neurology*. "Coexisting vitamin B12 deficiency might aggravate MS or impair recovery from MS."[28]

B3 (Niacin) Lowers Cholesterol Levels

In the 1950s, Abram Hoffer, M.D., discovered that niacin could be an effective treatment for some types of schizophrenia. He was also the first to recognize that the niacin form of vitamin B3 reduces blood cholesterol levels. (Conversely, while the niacinamide form of B3 helps some schizophrenics, it does not lower cholesterol.) Since then, more than 2,000 articles have been published by other doctors and researchers confirming the role of niacin in preventing heart disease and describing how the vitamin works. In fact, standard cardiology textbooks now cite the benefits of niacin, noting that it lowers levels of the "bad" LDL cholesterol by 25 percent and VLDL cholesterol by 75 percent, while increasing levels of the "good HDL" cholesterol by 20 to 40 percent.[29] Other than a temporary flushing sensation, niacin is free of side effects for most people. On the other hand, prescription drugs commonly administered to reduce cholesterol levels may cause gallbladder disease.

Niacin is so good at lowering cholesterol that some pharmaceutical firms have tested their proprietary drugs with the vitamin and recommend that the two be used together. This approach enables a larger profit from a patented drug while niacin—which is inexpensive—does much of the cholesterol-lowering work.

One such study on niacin was completed by John Kane, M.D., and published in the *Journal of the American Medical Association*. Patients taking niacin and the drug colestipol showed a dramatic reduction in both cholesterol levels and heart lesions. On average, cholesterol levels were reduced by almost 40 percent. Using X-ray analysis, Dr. Kane determined that coronary artery constriction also decreased, though slightly. It's very possible that the usually progressive lesions, which eventually block blood flow through the coronary arteries, could have been reduced even further if the study had been extended.[30]

VITAMIN C

Vitamin C increases life span, reduces symptoms of the common cold, protects against cancer and heart disease, lowers blood pressure, and reduces diabetic complications.

Shortly after the discovery and isolation of vitamin C 60 years ago, there was a surge of research on the role of vitamin C in health. In the 1930s and 1940s, dozens of articles in medical journals around the world reported that vitamin C deficiency aggravated viral and bacterial infections, promoted cancerous growths, worsened allergies, hastened the development of cardiovascular diseases, and made both laboratory animals and people more susceptible to environmental toxins. Conversely, other studies described vitamin C's protective and therapeutic benefits. Today, otherwise sensible people still argue whether vitamin C is beneficial, dangerous, or a waste of money.

"Since I've been writing in this field (of vitamin C), I've had the support of scientists," said Linus Pauling, now a robust 92. "They say that I've been right so often that I'm probably right here too. It's the medical community that has been blind."

Lengthens Life Span

A major study published last year silenced many of Pauling's—and vitamin C's—critics. Headlines such as "Live Longer With Vitamin C"[31] and "Heftier Doses of Vitamin C Reduce Death Rates, UCLA Study Indicates"[32] told much of the story.

James Enstrom, Ph.D., of the School of Public Health, University of California, Los Angeles, analyzed a ten-year federal health survey of 11,348 people ages 25 to 74. Reporting his findings in the May 1992 *Epidemiology*, Enstrom found that men who consumed 300 mg of vitamin C daily from food *and supplements* suffered 41 percent fewer deaths during the ten-year period compared with men who obtained only a meager 50 mg of the vitamin from diet alone. In analyzing the results, Enstrom accounted for other lifestyle factors that might have also extended life span.[33]

Scientists increasingly believe that tallying the number of people who die at each specific age (e.g., 64, 65, 66, etc.) may be a better way to assess aging than the more widely used concept of an average life span (e.g., 70 years of age). So it was significant that Enstrom determined than the men consuming 300 mg of vitamin C lived approximately six years longer than the low-vitamin C group. Even a modest daily intake of 150 mg of vitamin C increased life span by two years.

The benefits of vitamin C were less dramatic for women, although Enstrom was not sure why. Women taking high doses of vitamin C suffered only 10 percent fewer deaths as a group. But regardless of sex, the incidence of heart disease decreased as vitamin C intake increased.

Asked about the study, Pauling pointed out that Enstrom compared three categories of subjects: "Those with rather low intake of vitamin C in foods, below the RDA; those who took high levels of vitamin C in their foods; and those who also took vitamin C supplements. This (last) group had half the death rate from heart disease and a 30 percent lower cancer death rate."

In his conclusion, Enstrom wrote that his findings "are consistent with the hypothesis that high levels of antioxidant vitamins (such as vitamins C, E, and A) increase the body's defense system against free radicals and reduce the risk of arteriosclerosis. . . . Even if increased vitamin C intake *per se* has only a small beneficial effect, the population impact could still be substantial because of the large variations in dietary vitamin C intake and the widespread use of vitamin C supplements."

Relieves Common Cold Symptoms

Pauling first promoted the health benefits of vitamin C in his 1970 book, *Vitamin C and the Common Cold.* More than 100 subsequent studies showed mixed benefits—sometimes the vitamin C helped, sometimes it didn't.

However, a recent look at the data confirms Pauling's thesis that vitamin C fights colds. Harri Hemilä, Ph.D., of the University of Helsinki, Finland, recently analyzed 32 studies that closely followed the methods used in Pauling's 1971 study. Thirty-one studies supported the use of vitamin C in treating colds, and the remaining one showed vitamin C to be no less effective than a placebo.

Hemilä's analysis indicated that supplemental vitamin C does not reduce the frequency of colds. "However, vitamin C has consistently decreased the duration of cold episodes and the severity of symptoms," he wrote in the *British Journal of Nutrition.*[34] "The biochemical explanation for the benefits may be based on the antioxidant property of vitamin C. In an infection, phagocytic leucocytes become activated and they produce oxidizing compounds which are released from the cell. By reacting with these antioxidants, vitamin C may decrease the inflammatory effects caused by them."

Hemilä also pointed out that "the level of intake derived from a normal or balanced diet may be insufficient for optimal body function." Effective daily doses often range from 4 to 8 *grams*—and sometimes even higher. He described one double-blind study in which patients were given 6 grams of vitamin C daily at the beginning of a cold. "The benefits were so obvious that the physician could recognize the subjects receiving the vitamin by their clinical progress," Hemilä related. "Therefore the double-blind study was terminated, and a less-well-controlled study was performed."

Prevents and Slows Cancer

During the 1970s, Pauling's interest shifted to cancer research, and he began collaborating with Ewan Cameron, M.D., a Scottish physician who explored whether vitamin C might benefit terminal cancer patients. Pauling and Cameron charted the progress of terminal patients given 10 grams of vitamin C daily, then compared them to similar cancer patients treated by other doctors with surgery, radiation, and chemotherapy at the Vale of Leven Hospital in Loch Lomondside, Scotland. On average, the cancer patients taking vitamin C lived seven times longer than those that didn't. In fact, a couple of these terminal patients had total remissions.[35,36]

Fukumi Morishiga, M.D., Ph.D., president of Nakamura Memorial Hospital in Fukuoka, Japan, obtained similar results by also giving cancer patients 10 grams of vitamin C daily. But far more dramatic results came from a study by Canadian psychiatrist Abram Hoffer, M.D., Ph.D., who found himself in the 1980s treating cancer patients for depression and anxiety.

Hoffer, of Victoria, B.C., intended to treat only the psychiatric consequences of his terminal cancer patients, who had been referred to him by other doctors. He gave the patients 12 grams of vitamin C, 800 IU of vitamin E, 500 mg B3, and large amounts of vitamin A, beta-carotene, the B-complex vitamins, selenium, and other minerals. Inadvertently, Hoffer successfully treated many of the cancers.

Pauling analyzed the patients, focusing on 134 treated between April 1988 and April 1989. Thirty-three decided not to follow the program and lived only an additional four to five months. In contrast, most of the 101 terminal patients treated with vitamins and minerals were still alive several years later. Based on their early response to treatment, Pauling projected that their life expectancy would be five to seven years—or 15 times longer than conventionally treated patients. "So many are still alive that it's hard to predict how long they'll live," he said.

Hoffer, who had begun treating a group of 30 cancer patients back in 1982, said in an interview that nine of those terminal patients are still alive—ten years later. Meanwhile, Pauling offered this advice: "At the first sign that cancer is developing, you should go on Hoffer's program. We were recommending this 14 years ago. Every cancer patient should start this program and stay on it for the rest of his life."[37]

Fights Heart Disease

Most recently Pauling's attention has focused on the role of vitamin C in preventing heart disease. In fact, he and collaborator Matthias Rath, M.D., may have finally elucidated the fundamental cause of heart disease: too much of a blood fat known as lipoprotein(a) and too little vitamin C.

Lipoprotein(a) was discovered in 1946. However, it wasn't until just a couple of years ago that Rath determined that the deposition of lipoprotein(a) on arterial walls laid the groundwork for more plaque to accumulate. Then, Rath and Pauling stumbled across something that was even more startling.

Virtually all animals produce lipoprotein(a), but those that manufacture their own vitamin C make only small quantities of lipoprotein(a). On the other hand, those animals that do not make their own vitamin C—such as people—make large amounts of lipoprotein(a). Pauling said the lipoprotein(a) is the body's attempt to make a salve-like substance to heal and strengthen damaged arteries when they don't obtain enough vitamin C. [38,39]

And what precipitates a heart attack? Sometimes the lipoprotein(a) builds up to the point of blocking an artery. That, according to Pauling, results from inadequate vitamin C intake. At other times, a tear in a blood vessel in the heart or brain triggers a heart attack or stroke. That, too, results from insufficient vitamin C, according to Pauling. Such a tear, he explained, is a sign of weak collagen, a tissue "cement" that depends on vitamin C. "The proper intake of vitamin C can prevent and control heart disease, should it develop," Pauling said.

Vitamin C can apparently reduce hypertension as well. In a brief review of six other studies on vitamin C and blood pressure, Harri Hemilä, Ph.D., of the University of Helsinki, Finland, wrote that numerous animal studies and small-scale human studies have found that vitamin C can lower blood pressure.

"Vitamin C . . . participates in a large number of enzymatic and nonenzymatic reactions in all tissues and vitamin status may well affect blood pressure, even though any specific biochemical mechanisms are not yet obvious. Vitamin C is a cheap and safe nutrient. . . ," he wrote in the *Journal of Hypertension*. [40]

Protects Diabetics

Conventional approaches to the treatment of diabetes stress the control of blood sugar levels, but they have been less successful in treating the disease's complications: earlier than average onset of heart disease, including high blood pressure, high cholesterol levels, and the breakage of tiny blood vessels in the eye, resulting in blindness.

One important, though underestimated, link between diabetes

and heart disease may be vitamin C. It is well established in medicine that inadequate vitamin C intake results in a tendency toward capillary fragility, such as in the retinopathy in eye disease.

Chemically, the structures of vitamin C and glucose are very similar and, in most animal species (not *Homo sapiens*, however), glucose is converted to vitamin C. This relationship between diabetes and inadequate vitamin C did not escape notice by Anthony Verlangieri, Ph.D., of the University of Mississippi.

In *Life Sciences*, Dr. Verlangieri reported that high blood sugar levels prevent vitamin C from being fully utilized by the body. He contends that glucose competes with vitamin C on the cellular level, preventing the vitamin from entering the body's cells. In other words, high glucose levels may prevent the body from using vitamin C efficiently. In fact, many diabetic complications, such as retinopathy or high cholesterol levels, are consistent with inadequate intake or poor utilization of vitamin C. Supplemental C may partly displace this glucose, thus offering protection against some diabetic complications.[41]

VITAMIN E

Vitamin E protects against heart disease, cancer, Parkinson's disease, and tardive dyskinesia.

Protects Against Heart Disease

By reporting in 1992 that high blood levels of iron were associated with heart disease, Jukka Salonen, M.D., of the University of Kuopio, Finland, made a strong case in support of the free-radical cause of heart disease. The reason, according to his article in *Circulation*, is that iron promotes free-radical oxidation of tissues in people, and animal studies have shown that it can cause heart disease in animals.[42]

This particular study by Salonen did not consider the protective role of vitamin E but, for the nutritionally wise, the conclusion was unmistakable: Just as iron promotes free radicals and oxidation, vitamin E protects against them. Even more striking, iron and vitamin E are nutritional antagonists, and many dieticians have for years recommended that supplements of them not be consumed at the same time. In other words, if you take too much iron, you may diminish the value of your vitamin E.[43]

Indeed, other well-designed studies have established a clear relationship between low levels of vitamin E and heart disease. Among the most significant were two major studies reported at the November 1992 meeting of the American Heart Association, held in New Orleans.

Both were conducted at Boston's Brigham and Women's Hospital and the Harvard School of Public Health. The Nurses Health Study followed 87,245 women ages 34 to 59 who were free of heart disease when the study began in 1980. Meanwhile, the Health Professionals Follow-up Study looked at 45,720 men ages 40 to 75 with no history of heart disease as of 1986.

Seventeen percent of the nurses took vitamin E supplements at some time between 1980 and 1988, according to researcher Meir Stampfer, M.D., an associate professor at the Harvard School of Public Health. During that time, 552 cases of heart attack were diagnosed in the test group. After adjusting for age, smoking, obesity, exercise, and other risk factors, Stampfer and his colleagues found that the nurses taking vitamin E supplements had only two-thirds (64 percent) the risk of cardiovascular disease, compared with those not taking the vitamin supplement. Women who took vitamin E for more than two years had an even lower risk of developing heart disease, only 54 percent. Taking vitamin E more consistently for longer periods of time might have reduced their heart disease risk further.

The study of male health workers yielded similar results. After adjusting for major cardiovascular disease risk factors, researchers determined that the men taking vitamin E for more than two years had a 26 percent lower risk of heart disease than those not taking the vitamin, according to Eric Rimm, Sc.D., a research associate in the Harvard School of Public Health.

"I'm skeptical by nature, but I was even more skeptical going into this study," Stampfer said in an interview during the Heart Association meeting. "It just didn't seem plausible that a simple maneuver like taking vitamin E would have such a profound effect. So even though there was really a sound scientific basis for the hypothesis that antioxidant vitamins can reduce heart disease, I expected to show that this was not in fact a true association."

The protective effect was seen in people taking at least 100 international units of vitamin E per day, even after both research teams adjusted for vitamin C and beta-carotene intake. No benefits were seen from vitamin E obtained in diet alone.

An earlier study by R. A. Riemersma, Ph.D., of the University of Edinburgh, questioned 6,000 Scottish men about their symptoms of angina pectoris, a chest pain caused by inadequate oxygen in the heart muscle. Riemersma found that men with low vitamin E intake were twice as likely to suffer from angina as those with high levels, according to an article in *Vitamin E: Biochemistry and Health Implications, Annals of the New York Academy of Sciences.* In a later analysis of the data, published in *Lancet,* Riemersma found that levels of vitamin E, beta-carotene and vitamin C, also antioxidants, protected against angina.[44,45]

Why does vitamin E help the heart? Three other studies explain. In a study on monkeys, Anthony Verlangieri, Ph.D., of the University of Mississippi, found that vitamin E slowed—and, at times, even reversed—fatty build-ups on the walls of arteries. Verlangieri gave six monkeys a typical laboratory diet, six others a diet laced with cholesterol and lard, and six others a similar high-fat diet but with vitamin E supplements. After three years, the monkeys eating their typical diet showed no sign of heart disease. Meanwhile, ultrasound tests on the monkeys eating a high-fat diet showed an 87 percent blockage of the carotid artery. The monkeys on a high-fat diet plus vitamin E had only an average 61 percent blockage of the carotid artery, according to an article in the *Journal of the American College of Nutrition.*[46] In other words, while a sound diet may be the best preventive for heart disease, vitamin E offers substantial protection against a high-fat diet.

Ishwarlal Jialal, M.D., of the University of Texas Southwestern Medical Center, Dallas, has shown that vitamin E prevents cholesterol from being oxidized and, in effect, "going bad." In a study of 24 volunteer subjects, Jialal gave 12 men 800 IU of vitamin E per day and 12 others a placebo for three months. In analyzing blood samples, he found that the vitamin E supplements increased the level of this vitamin in the blood and in the low-density lipoprotein, preventing its oxidation. Low-density lipoprotein, or LDL, is considered the "bad" form of cholesterol, and high levels of it are closely associated with heart disease.[47]

Finally, platelet adhesion, or unusual stickiness of blood platelet cells, is also a factor in heart disease, particularly in the clots that trigger heart attacks. Dr. J. Jandak, writing in the journal *Blood,* reported that platelet adhesion decreased by 75 percent when patients took 200 IU of vitamin E a day for two weeks. Even better, the patients' platelet stickiness decreased by an amazing 82 percent after they took 400 IU of vitamin E for two weeks.[48,49]

Protects Against Cancer

As an antioxidant nutrient, vitamin E also protects against cancer. Gloria Gridley, Ph.D., and her colleagues at the National Cancer Institute analyzed data from more than 1,100 people with oral cancer and compared their use of dietary supplements with 1,300 healthy subjects. Gridley found that supplements of vitamin A, B, and C decreased the risk of oral cancer, but vitamin E cut the risk in half.

"To the authors' knowledge, this is the first epidemiological study to show a reduced oral cancer risk with vitamin E use," Gridley and her associates wrote in the *American Journal of Epidemiology.*[50] "Although it is not clear that the lower risk among consumers of vitamin E supplements is due to the vitamin per se, the findings are consistent with experimental evidence and should prompt further research on the role of vitamin E and other micronutrients as inhibitors of oral and pharyngeal cancer."

Interviewed for a news story in the *Journal of the National Cancer Institute,* Gridley was quoted as saying, "It appeared that all the separate vitamins had a protective effect when, in fact, it was all being driven by vitamin E." As it turned out, virtually everyone who took vitamin E also took at least one other supplement.[51]

However, the amount of vitamin E typically found in a multivitamin supplement—30 IU—may not be enough. "The reduced risk was only for those who took a separate vitamin E, although we didn't ask about dose," Gridley said.

A long-term epidemiological study, begun in 1968, found that vitamin E protects against virtually all types of cancers. Paul Knekt, Ph.D., a researcher at Finland's Social Insurance Institution, was the chief investigator in the study of 36,000 Finnish citizens. Knekt and his co-researchers followed the health of these people and came to the conclusion that "high vitamin E intake protects against cancer."

In one analysis of the data, Knekt looked at 21,000 men who were initially free of cancer. After ten years, 453 of the men had developed the disease. Regardless of the type or location of the cancer, these men had substantially lower vitamin E levels than comparable healthy men. On the other hand, "a high serum alpha-tocopherol (vitamin E) level was associated with a reduced risk of cancer," Knekt wrote in the *American Journal of Epidemiology.*[52]

In another breakdown of the data, Dr. Knekt analyzed the diets and medical histories of 15,000 Finnish women. Eight years after the study began, 313 of the women had developed cancers. Those who had the lowest blood levels of vitamin E were 50 percent more likely to develop epithelial cancers. Although hormone (estrogen)-related cancers were not associated with low vitamin E intake alone, they did correspond to inadequate intake of vitamin E and selenium.[53]

Combats Crippling Neurological Disorders

Some of the most dramatic findings relate to vitamin E and the health of the brain. Numerous recent studies have found that the vitamin can combat such devastating neurological disorders as tardive dyskinesia and Parkinson's disease.

R. J. Sokol, Ph.D., writing in the *Annual Review of Nutrition*, pointed out "that vitamin E is an essential nutrient necessary for the optimal development and maintenance of the integrity and function of the human nervous system and skeletal muscle."[54]

The brain seems to be particularly sensitive to vitamin E deficiency because the membranes of brain cells are rich in polyunsaturated fatty acids, prone to free-radical oxidation, according to C. P. LeBel, Ph.D., writing in *Biochemical and Biophysical Research Communications*. He believes that vitamin E is stored in brain cell membranes specifically to slow the formation of free radicals.[55]

Perhaps not surprisingly, then, vitamin E can improve the condition of people suffering from tardive dyskinesia, characterized by involuntary movements of the facial muscles, arms, and legs. Although tardive dyskinesia can arise spontaneously, it is more common among patients taking anti-psychotic drugs, which promote free radicals. Jean Lud Cadet, M.D., of the Neurological Institute at New York's Columbia University and James Lohi, M.D., of the psychiatry department of the University of California, San Diego, used vitamin E to treat 15 patients with severe tardive dyskinesia. Almost half of the patients improved, the doctors reported in *Vitamin E: Biochemistry and Health Implications, Annals of the New York Academy of Sciences*.[56]

Vitamin E may also benefit patients suffering from Parkinson's disease, characterized by muscular weakness, tremors, and partial facial paralysis. Stanley Fahn, M.D., a neurologist at the Columbia University College of Physicians and Surgeons, found that vitamin E's antioxidant properties delay the progression of Parkinson's disease and reduce its severity. He was one of many physicians presenting papers at "Vitamin E: Biochemistry and Health Implications," an international conference sponsored by the New York Academy of Sciences, Oct. 31–Nov. 2, 1988.

At the vitamin E conference, Fahn described a group of 14 patients who had not yet begun receiving L-dopa, a drug that reduces Parkinson's symptoms but also has side effects. "The patients on antioxidants went 2.5 years longer before they needed levodopa to treat their Parkinson's disease symptoms, suggesting that antioxidants may be useful in slowing down the progression of Parkinson's disease," he said.[57]

In fact, L. I. Golbe, M.D., who conducted another study on vitamin E and Parkinson's disease, believes that daily intake of vitamin E may delay the onset of Parkinson's by as much as 50 percent compared with untreated patients. "Our data are consistent with the hypothesis that vitamin E, as an antioxidant, may have prophylactic value against Parkinson's disease," he wrote in *Archives of Neurology*.[58]

GETTING THE MOST OUT OF YOUR MINERALS

CALCIUM

Calcium prevents and serves as an effective treatment for high blood pressure. Supplements can also help prevent bone loss.

Lowers Blood Pressure

Researchers have recently demonstrated that an ample intake of calcium can often prevent high blood pressure. Their findings add to the evidence indicating that calcium supplements can effectively treat hypertension.

James Dwyer, Ph.D., of the Southern California School of Medicine, analyzed the calcium intake of 6,634 men and women who were free of hypertension when they began participating in a 13-year epidemiological study. He found that people who consumed at least 1 gram of calcium daily had a 12 percent lower risk of developing high blood pressure compared with those obtaining less of the mineral. Dwyer presented his findings at the November 1992 meeting of the American Heart Association in New Orleans, according to a report in *Science News*.[59]

An estimated 63 million people in the United States suffer from hypertension, increasing their risk of other heart diseases, stroke, and kidney disease. If your blood pressure is approximately 120/80 (described as "120 over 80"), it's normal. On the other hand, if your blood pressure is in the range of 160/95 to 180/115, it is moderately high. And if it is higher than 180/115, it is markedly elevated.

People under age 40 seemed to have even greater benefits from a high-calcium diet. It reduced their likelihood of developing hypertension by 25 percent. And, for some unknown reason, thin people eating a high-calcium diet had an 18 percent reduction in blood pressure risk, compared with heavier people.

Dwyer's research echoes the work of David McCarron, M.D., who proposed in 1984 that too little calcium, rather than too much salt, might be a major cause of high blood pressure. McCarron, a kidney and hypertension specialist at Oregon Health Sciences University in Portland, reported in the journal *Science* that low dietary intakes of calcium, potassium, vitamins A and C, and even sodium (as in sodium chloride, or salt) were associated with hypertension.[60]

The work of other researchers and clinicians has tended to support the calcium hypothesis. For example, Komei Sato, M.D. and his colleagues at Hidaka Hospital and Kobe University School of Medicine in Japan found that calcium supplements prevented increases in blood pressure among patients on a high-salt diet, according to an article published in the journal *Hypertension*. Based on cellular changes, he concluded that the calcium lowered blood pressure by reducing the amount of sodium retained by the body.[61]

Calcium supplements also appear to prevent gestational hypertension, a rise in blood pressure during pregnancy. José Belizán, M.D., of the Rosarino Center for Prenatal Studies in Rosario, Argentina, and José Villar, M.D., of the World Health organization in Geneva, Switzerland, studied 1,194 pregnant women, half of whom were given daily calcium supplements. "Pregnant women who receive calcium supplementation after the 20th week of pregnancy have a reduced risk of hypertension disorders of pregnancies," the doctors reported in the *New England Journal of Medicine*.

Among the women taking calcium supplements, only 9.8 percent had hypertension, compared with 14.8 percent of the women receiving placebos.[62]

In another study, two physicians found that the blood pressure of pregnant women influences the blood pressure of their babies. Stephen McGarvey, M.D., and Stephan Zinner, M.D., of Brown University, looked at the eating habits of 212 pregnant women. They found that higher blood pressures were associated with lower intakes of three minerals. Writing in *Hypertension*, they reported that the "maternal prenatal intakes of potassium, calcium, and perhaps magnesium, influence infant blood pressure throughout the first year of life."[63]

In an article in the *American Journal of Clinical Nutrition*, McCarron recently stated that a daily intake of 700 to 800 mg of calcium—roughly equivalent to the recommended daily allowance for adults—would likely protect against high blood pressure. However, Dr. McCarron noted that this amount may vary from person to person depending on general dietary habits, lifestyle, and genetics—and that many people likely need far higher amounts of calcium.[64]

McCarron has argued that physicians need to take an "integrated" view of the role of sodium, calcium, potassium, and other minerals in the control of hypertension. "For example, treatment of 'sodium chloride sensitivity' in some humans might be more effectively approached by correcting dietary deficiencies of either potassium or calcium than by restricting dietary sodium chloride," he wrote in *Hypertension*.[65]

"Nutrients are not consumed in isolation but as interactive constituents of total diet. . . . We have the clues at hand to appreciate that simply focusing our health policy on lower sodium chloride intake to both prevent and to treat high blood pressure is setting a course of limited effectiveness," he added.

Supplements Prevent Bone Loss

The role of calcium deficiency in osteoporosis has been recognized—and debated needlessly—for decades. The most common medical treatment for osteoporosis in postmenopausal women is estrogen, but the hormone increases cancer risk. To put the arguments to rest, Drs. J. A. Kanis and R. Passmore, writing in the *British Medical Journal*, keenly observed, "Even if calcium were only

1 percent more effective than placebo (dummy pill) in reducing the incidence of fractures, it would prevent more than 1,000 fractures a year in Britain."[66]

It was a sage comment. Since 1988, 27 of 43 medical studies showed that calcium supplements helped prevent or reduce bone loss. And in February 1993, Ian Reid, M.D., of the University of Aukland, New Zealand, announced what may be the most conclusive evidence so far. Reid studied 122 women who had gone through menopause at least three years before. They were getting about 750 mg of calcium daily, already more than the typical American woman obtains from her diet. Half of the women in the study were given another 1,000 mg calcium daily, while the others received a placebo.

Writing in the *New England Journal of Medicine*, Reid explained that the women receiving the placebo lost about one percent of bone yearly. Meanwhile, women taking the calcium supplements lost only about one-half percent of bone, according to Reid.[67] In an editorial in the same issue, Robert Heaney, M.D., of Creighton University, recommended that women take 1,000 to 1,500 mg of calcium and 400 to 800 IU of vitamin D (which helps calcium absorption) "without waiting for more information."[68]

In a review of the medical literature on osteoporosis and calcium deficiency, Heaney and Christopher Nordin, M.D., of Adelaide, South Australia, argued that the disease could be prevented through increased consumption of milk products or calcium supplements. Writing in the *British Medical Journal*, they pointed out that "the evidence suggests that a significant component of the osteoporosis which affects so many postmenopausal women in the West is attributable to a relative or absolute inadequacy of calcium intake and hence is potentially and easily preventable."[69]

Adding to the evidence is the work of Miriam Nelson, M.D., of the Human Nutrition Research Center on Aging at Tufts University, Boston. Nelson studied 36 postmenopausal women and found that both calcium-rich dairy products and exercise prevented the bone loss characteristic of osteoporosis. However, they found that the calcium and the exercise helped different bones.

Writing in the *American Journal of Clinical Nutrition*, Nelson reported that a vigorous 50-minute walk four times a week increased trabecular bone mass in the spine by 0.5 percent. At the same time, sedentary women in the study had a 7 percent loss of bone mass in the spine. Calcium supplementation had no effect on this particular bone.[70]

In contrast, calcium intake—and not exercise—affected the density of the thighbone. Nelson determined that thighbone density increased by 2 percent among women drinking a milk-based high-calcium supplement. Among women not taking the supplement, thighbone density decreased by 1.1 percent.

MAGNESIUM

Magnesium controls arrhythmias and reduces the risk of death following a heart attack. It also lowers cholesterol levels and reduces many complications of diabetes.

Prevents Arrhythmias

Supplements of magnesium can prevent many types of arrhythmias. However, during a potentially fatal attack, or immediately after a heart attack, oral supplements work too slowly. Increasingly, emergency-room physicians and cardiologists are giving patients intravenous solutions of magnesium to reduce their risk of death.

For example, injections of the mineral magnesium reduced heart attack deaths by one fourth, according to a study published in the British journal *Lancet*. Kent L. Woods, M.D., of the University of Leicester, England, reported that magnesium's benefits were as good as aspirin and the more highly touted clot-dissolving drugs streptokinase and TPA. "Intravenous magnesium sulfate is a simple, safe, and widely applicable treatment," he wrote.[71]

Woods conducted a well-controlled double-blind study on 2,316 patients suffering from myocardial infarction. The patients received intravenous magnesium sulfate or a simple saline (salt water) solution. After 28 days—an especially high-risk time for heart attack victims—only 7.8 percent of the patients given magnesium died, compared with 10.3 percent of those receiving conventional treatments alone. Looked at a different way, an additional 25 people per thousand survived their heart attacks because of the magnesium.

Most researchers believe that magnesium works by stimulating the sodium-potassium-ATPase pump, which regulates much of the heart's electrical activity. Others believe that many of the mineral's cardiac benefits are related to its anti-clotting properties or "direct protective action" on the heart muscle, according to Woods.

One of the most significant magnesium studies was conducted by L. F. Smith, M.D., of the University of Leicester, England, and involved the treatment of 200 patients hospitalized after suffering a heart attack. Reporting his findings in the *International Journal of Cardiology*, Smith found that magnesium reduced the incidence of arrhythmias and sudden death syndrome by more than 50 percent.[72]

Most recently, Leszek Ceremuzynski, M.D., of Warsaw's Grochowski Hospital, reported that magnesium prevented ventricular tachycardia (rapid heartbeat originating in the ventricles) in heart-attack victims. "The most striking finding was a much lower incidence of VT (ventricular tachycardia) in patients given magnesium *supplements*," he wrote in the *American Heart Journal*. Only seven, or 28 percent, of the 25 patients given magnesium had arrhythmias, compared with more than three-fourths of a comparable group of people who did not receive magnesium supplements.[73]

Sometimes arrhythmias are caused by drugs doctors use to treat other types of heart disease. For example, the heart stimulant digitalis works by blocking the sodium-potassium-ATPase cellular pump. While digitalis can extend the life of people suffering from congestive heart failure, it does interfere with the normal roles of magnesium and potassium. One consequence is that heart cells become more excitable and prone to arrhythmias.

Digitalis "intoxication" can cause arrhythmias and premature ventricular contractions (PVCs). In fact, patients taking digitalis are twice as likely to be deficient in magnesium as potassium, according to cardiologists Andre Keren, M.D., and Dan Tzivoni, M.D., of Jerusalem, Israel. Writing in the journal *Pacing and Clinical Electrophysiology*, they noted that "Potassium replacement in these patients has to be accompanied by concomitant magnesium therapy for correction of intracellular potassium deficit," they explained.[74]

Diuretics and thiazides, drugs given to treat heart failure and high blood pressure, rapidly deplete magnesium and potassium. "While potassium loss is routinely corrected, magnesium replacement is usually neglected," Keren and Tzivoni pointed out. "Among 297 patients with congestive heart failure who received diuretics, hypomagnesemia was present in 37 percent, and low skeletal muscle magnesium was found in 43 percent of cases."

Helps Diabetics

Magnesium may be one of the most underrated nutrients in the treatment of diabetes and its complications. Many medical studies have shown that magnesium deficiency may be a factor in high blood pressure among nondiabetics. At the University of Southern California in Los Angeles, Samuel Malayan, M.D., has extended this research by linking low magnesium blood levels to high blood pressure in Type II diabetics. The association between inadequate magnesium and high blood pressure is significant because elevated blood pressure increases the risk of kidney disease in both diabetics and nondiabetics.

At a 1990 American Health Association meeting in Baltimore, Malayan reported that magnesium probably lowered blood pressure by relaxing constricted blood vessels. He gave seven hypertensive diabetics daily doses of 260 mg of magnesium. Six weeks later, their average blood pressure had dropped from 157/96 to 128/77, according to a report in *Science News*.[75]

According to Arshag Mooradian, M.D., of the Veterans Administration Medical Center in Sepulveda, Calif., magnesium is needed for glucose transport in the body and is part of numerous enzymes involved in glucose metabolism. In addition, magnesium also seems to play a role in the release of insulin.

Magnesium deficiency is linked to two common diabetic complications, according to Mooradian. One is retinopathy, the deterioration of tiny blood vessels in the eyes that can lead to blindness. In a study cited by Dr. Mooradian, patients with severe diabetic retinopathy had lower blood levels of magnesium than did diabetics with minimal retinal disease.[76]

The other complication closely linked to magnesium deficiency in diabetics is an increased risk of heart disease. Burton Altura, Ph.D., of the State University of New York, Brooklyn, fed cholesterol-laced meals to several groups of rabbits which are highly susceptible to artery-clogging atherosclerosis. One group of rabbits received a normal amount of magnesium. A second group received only 60 percent of their recommended daily allowance for magnesium, and a third group received three times the usual allowance for magnesium. A fourth group of rabbits was given cholesterol-free meals.

While only the cholesterol-fed rabbits developed atherosclerotic deposits in the heart, the magnesium-deficient rabbits developed the thickest deposits. Those with the highest magnesium intake developed the fewest and thinnest deposits.[77]

In a study of 430 patients over 12 weeks, R. B. Singh, M.D., chief cardiologist and professor of clinical nutrition at the Moradabad Medical Hospital and Research Center, India, confirmed that a magnesium-rich diet decreased levels of total blood cholesterol, the "bad" low-density-lipoprotein cholesterol, and triglyceride by just over 10 percent. Discussing his findings in the journal *Magnesium*, he added an interesting observation: "There is some evidence that high dietary fat can inhibit the absorption of magnesium, and that the inhibition is more intense with saturated than polyunsaturated fat."[78]

CHROMIUM

Chromium lowers cholesterol and lengthens life span.

Chromium, a mineral known to be essential for managing blood sugar, may also extend life span, according to a study announced at the annual meeting of the American Aging Association, October 9, 1992, in San Francisco.

Gary Evans, Ph.D., of Bemidji State University in Minnesota, supplemented the diets of laboratory rats with chromium picolinate, chromium nicotinate, and chromium chloride. After 41 months, all of the rats had died except for 80 percent of those fed chromium picolinate. These rats lived about one year longer than the others, a 36 percent increase in lifespan. While extrapolations to humans may not be scientific, the equivalent life extension in people would be from about 75 years to 102.

Because high blood sugar levels appear to have a role in aging, Evans measured the rats' blood sugar and glycated hemoglobin levels. Glycation is a measure of how sugar alters proteins, and it may be the basis for many of the changes that characterize aging.

Since 1935, researchers have known that caloric restriction can dramatically extend the life span of rodents and reduce the risk of degenerative diseases. This study demonstrated such life extension without caloric restriction.

"Chromium picolinate enhances insulin function and may therefore produce the same glucose-lowering benefits as underfeeding, but without restriction of calorie intake," said Evans.

In an earlier study, published in the January 1990 *Western Journal of Medicine*, he wrote that a daily 200 mcg supplement of the mineral lowered total cholesterol, LDL cholesterol, and apolipoprotein B (the principal fraction of LDL) in a group of 28 subjects.[79]

SELENIUM

Selenium, which works with vitamin E, protects the heart and fights cancer.

Selenium is a powerful antioxidant that increases the benefits of vitamin E and glutathione peroxidase, two other key antioxidants. According to recent research by investigators of the University of Illinois, Urbana, and the University of Wisconsin, Madison, selenium deficiency can reduce the heart's antioxidant defenses.

"Selenium is not the only factor which determines myocardial susceptibility to oxidative stress," explained L. L. Ji, Ph.D., in the *Journal of the American College of Nutrition.* "Indeed, vitamin E is believed to play an important role in this regard. It has been demonstrated that when animals suffer from selenium and vitamin E double deficiencies, the oxidative damage observed is more severe than with deficiency of either antioxidant alone."[80]

Meanwhile, Diane Birt, Ph.D., of the University of Nebraska Medical Center in Omaha, has pointed out that the incidence of cancer decreases as selenium intake increases. She added that selenium's anticancer benefits "appear to be the strongest" when it is taken soon after the cancer develops, "although evidence suggests that (selenium's) effects on later stages of cancer may also be important."[81]

In a study of more than 15,000 Finnish women, Paul Knekt, Ph.D., found that estrogen-related cancers correlated to poor intake of both selenium and vitamin E. In fact, women with low consumption of these two nutrients had a risk of breast cancer 10 times the average.[82] Inadequate amounts of selenium and vitamin E also increased the risk of cancers of the upper gastrointestinal tract, according to Knekt.

In the *International Journal of Cancer,* Knekt pointed out that "we found higher serum selenium and serum vitamin E levels to be associated with a lower risk of cancer of the upper gastrointestinal tract. . . . The association was stronger for men than for women. The results are in line with the hypothesis that high selenium and vitamin E intake protect against some cancers caused by dietary factors."[83]

ZINC

Used as a lozenge, zinc fights colds and sore throats.

Fights Colds

In the late 1970s, William Halcomb, M.D. and one of his patients accidentally discovered that zinc, taken as a lozenge, reduced cold symptoms and the overall length of the infection—if the zinc was taken within a day or two of the cold's onset. To confirm the value of zinc lozenges, Dr. Halcomb and George Eby conducted a controlled, double-blind study with the results analyzed by Dr. Donald Davis of the Clayton Foundation Biochemical Institute, University of Texas, Austin.

In this first study, reported in the journal *Antimicrobial Agents and Chemotherapy*, Dr. Halcomb gave 146 people either a 180-mg zinc gluconate tablet (containing 23 mg or elemental zinc) or a placebo (inert tablet) within the first couple days of a cold. The patients were instructed to suck on the tablets for at least 10 minutes, allowing the zinc to dissolve and bathe the throat. They dissolved two tablets initially and then dissolved another every two hours. Adults took no more than 12 tablets daily, and children took fewer.[84]

Halcomb, Eby, and Davis found that large numbers of zinc-treated subjects became well within hours: 11 percent within 12 hours and 22 percent within 24 hours, while none of the people taking the inert tablets became well. On the average, subjects who had taken the zinc recovered completely in less than four days. Those who took the placebo averaged 11 days for recovery.

Since then, studies on the use of zinc in fighting colds and sore throats have shown mixed benefits. Sometimes the zinc helped, sometimes it had no effect.

One reason, according to John C. Godfrey, Ph.D., may be that some of the zinc formulations contained additives that, when combined with saliva, inactivated the zinc. So, Godfrey and B. Conant Sloane, M.D., of the Dartmouth College Health Service, used a different form of zinc—zinc gluconate-glycine—in a radomized, placebo-controlled double-blind study. They treated 73 men and women between the ages of 18 and 40 with either 23.7-mg zinc supplements or a comparably astringent tannic-acid-based placebo.

"Patients' symptoms first appeared 1.34 days prior to entry to the study in both groups," wrote the researchers in the *Journal of International Medical Research*. Disappearance of symptoms occurred aft.r an additional 4.9 days for zinc-treated patients versus 6.1 days for placebo-treated patients. A difference was noted in the efficacy of treatment if it was started 1 day after symptom onset: cold duration was [only] an additional 4.3 days in zinc-treated patients compared with 9.2 days for placebo-treated patients."[85]

The researchers used the strict criterion of "complete disappearance of all symptoms" to define the end of the cold. The symptoms most affected were cough, nasal drainage, and congestion.

"The effects observed in the present study indicate that there may be a one- to two-day 'window of opportunity' for treatment with ZGG (zinc gluconate-glycine) before the common cold takes hold," wrote the researchers. "It could be determined from further studies whether cold symptoms would last an even shorter time if ZGG treatment were begun on the day of symptom onset."

Godfrey and Sloane hypothesized that zinc worked in two ways. First, the mineral appeared to function as an antiviral agent, a role documented by previous studies. Second, zinc also seemed to have some benefits by acting as an astringent on throat tissues. For this reason, the researchers matched the astringency of the placebo to the zinc lozenge. They did concede that "it was not surprising to discover that the placebo appeared to have some activity, although significantly less than ZGG."

Helps Memory

Harold Sandstead, M.D., of the University of Texas, Galveston, gave 30-mg supplements of iron or zinc to 26 women deficient in these minerals. After taking the supplements, the women increased their scores on the Wechsler Memory test by an average of 10 percent—and some by up to 20 percent. However, women who took both minerals did not improve their scores, apparently because the minerals interfered with each other.

Speaking at the April 1990 meeting of the Federation of American Societies for Experimental Biology in Atlanta, Dr. Sanstead noted that iron and zinc also improved memory in different ways. Iron improved short-term recall of verbal information, whereas zinc improved the ability to associate word pairs, according to a report in *Science News*.[86]

HOW VITAMINS AND MINERALS WORK TOGETHER

By now, you can see that vitamins and minerals have impressive roles in maintaining and restoring health. While all such micronutrients have their individual benefits, the reality is that they ultimately work together—and, occasionally, against each other. This means that taking vitamin and mineral supplements demands more than simply reading labels. It requires a healthy dose of homework to make sure they work for you.

David L. Watts, D.C., Ph.D., of Addison, Texas, likens these nutritional interrelationships to the intermeshing gears of a bicycle. Because all of the "gears"—nutrients—are either directly or indirectly connected, a change in one may affect others. By using the findings of more than 150,000 mineral analyses on patients around the country, Dr. Watts has made sense of the complex interactions among vitamins and minerals, so people can use supplements to their greatest advantage without messing up the gears.[87]

Why are vitamin-mineral interactions important? First, the right combination of nutrients can promote nutrient synergism—that is, help vitamins and minerals work together. Second, the right combination of nutrients can minimize nutrient antagonism—in other words, reduce the likelihood that nutrients will work against each other.

For the most part, nutrients work in unison. Consider the positive interactions of a few of the vitamins:

- Vitamins C and E help the body use vitamin A.
- Vitamins A, C, and B12 help the body use vitamin E.

Likewise, synergisms exist among minerals. Consider these examples.

- Magnesium promotes the body's use of potassium.
- Calcium, magnesium, and phosphorus work together to build and maintain bone.

Similarly, synergisms exist between vitamins and minerals, adding to the complexity. Examples:

- Both vitamin D and calcium are needed to correct many bone diseases, including osteoporosis and rickets.
- Copper, vitamins C, B6, and A are needed along with iron to help a person fully recover from an iron deficiency.
- Zinc is needed to correct a vitamin A deficiency.

The problem is that vitamins and minerals can also work against each other, leading to nutritional imbalances. When a person requires two antagonistic nutrients, such as iron and vitamin E, the solution may be as simple as taking them at different times of the day.

There are other common nutritional antagonisms. Among them:

- High calcium or copper intake depresses zinc.
- Vitamin B1 reduces uptake of vitamin B12.
- Surprisingly, vitamins A and D are antagonistic.

APPLYING YOUR KNOWLEDGE OF NUTRIENT INTERACTIONS

The charts included in this book offer detailed information describing how vitamins and minerals interact. The obvious question is, "How do I use this information without getting totally confused?"

If you're in generally good health and planning to take only a multi-vitamin and multi-mineral supplement, you don't have to be very concerned about nutrient interactions. Although such supplements vary somewhat in the amounts and ratios of the vitamins and minerals they contain, they do strive for balance.

On the other hand, if you suffer from a specific condition, odds are that your nutritional profile is already unbalanced—and should be corrected. In addition, vitamin and mineral interactions become much more important when you take megadoses to treat specific conditions.

Watts leans heavily on the research of the late Melvin Page, M.D., who categorized many diseases as either sympathetic or parasympathetic, referring to the body's nervous systems. If you are a hard-driving, impatient, Type-A personality, you may be at greater risk of developing what Page called sympathetic diseases. These include: anxiety, rheumatoid arthritis, histamine allergies, high blood pressure, hyperthyroidism, Hodgkin's disease, leukemia, bacterial infections, multiple sclerosis, peptic or duodenal ulcers, and juvenile-onset diabetes. According to Watts, these diseases tend to be associated with high levels of one or more stimulatory nutrients: phosphorus, sodium, potassium, iron, manganese, selenium, and vitamins A, E, B1, B6, and folic acid.

If you have a laid-back, passive, Type-B personality, you may be at greater risk of developing parasympathetic diseases, including: osteoarthritis, low-histamine allergies, asthma, AIDS, anorexia, premenstrual syndrome, Candida infections, gastric ulcers, and adult-onset diabetes. People with these diseases tend to have high levels of sedative nutrients, including calcium, magnesium, zinc, copper, chromium, and vitamins D, B2, B12, and choline.

Describing these two categories is not to say that high levels of these nutrients cause these diseases. Rather, unusually high levels of these nutrients are often consistent with other symptoms of the diseases. Reducing their levels—or improving the ratios between nutrients—may help normalize the many biochemical reactions that have gone awry during the illness.

As you may have already surmised, treatment should (at least in part) restore a more balanced nutritional profile. In other words, if your nutritional profile is unbalanced, balanced supplements won't correct it. You need an unbalanced supplement that mirrors your nutritional profile. For example, if your nutritional profile shows high levels of stimulatory nutrients, you may need to take sedative nutrients to achieve a balance. Conversely, if your nutritional profile shows high levels of sedative nutrients, you may need to take stimulatory nutrients.

How do you determine your nutritional profile? Recognizing whether you are a Type A or Type B personality may give you a clue. In addition, if you suffer from a sympathetic disease, such as rheumatoid arthritis, that may be another clue. For a more accurate determination, ask your doctor for a hair analysis of mineral levels.

Hair analysis measures mineral levels over several weeks and may be more informative than blood tests, which measure minerals on a particular day. While one hair analysis may provide a wealth of information, arranging for such a test two to four times a year will show changes, particularly if you want to know how corrective supplements change your nutritional profile. While a hair analysis cannot measure vitamin levels, the mineral levels may indirectly provide some information, based on the known synergisms and antagonisms between vitamins and minerals.

By knowing your nutritional profile and how vitamins and minerals interact, you can combine them for maximum benefit. For example, vitamin E might be helpful to people with heart disease or benign breast cysts. However, the addition of selenium makes vitamin E much more effective. Likewise, while iron supplements may help people with iron-deficiency anemia, additional vitamin C aids iron metabolism.

OTHER INTERACTIONS YOU SHOULD KNOW ABOUT

Prescription or over-the-counter drugs you purchase may also interact with vitamins and minerals in a variety of ways. Sometimes, nutritional supplements will increase or decrease the effect of drugs. At other times, drugs will decrease the benefits of vitamins and minerals. If you take prescription medicines, it is worthwhile keeping in mind how they interact with vitamins and minerals. The following information is an overview. For more details, consult *The Complete Guide to Vitamins, Minerals & Supplements,* by H. Winter Griffith, M.D.[88]

Vitamin A: Antacids, cholestyramine, and colestipol may decrease absorption of vitamin A. Anticoagulants taken with vitamin A increase risk of bleeding.

Vitamin C: Salicylates, sulfa drugs, and tetracyclines reduce the benefits of vitamin C.

Vitamin E: Vitamin E may reduce insulin requirements in diabetics. Use it with extreme caution in people with rheumatic heart disease. Antacids, cholestyramine, cholestipol, mineral oil, and sucralfate may decrease absorption of vitamin E. Vitamin E may reduce the effectiveness of iron supplements, particularly in people with iron-deficiency anemia. Combined with anticoagulants, such as coumarin, aspirin, or chamomile tea, vitamin E may increase bleeding.

Vitamin B Complex: Vitamin B1 seems to increase the effect of muscle-relaxant drugs given during surgery. Vitamin B2 may turn urine yellow, but it poses no harm. Antidepressants decrease the effect of B2. Niacin combined with beta-blocker medications may lower blood pressure to dangerous levels. Hydrazides, penicillamine, adrenocorticoids, and cyclosporine may increase requirements for vitamin B6. Vitamin B6 may reduce the effect of L-dopa. Very high doses of vitamin B6 may cause peripheral neuropathy; deficiencies may have the same effect. Folic acid may mask symptoms of a vitamin B12 deficiency. Cortisone drugs and oral contraceptives reduce benefits of folic acid. Low doses of pantothenic acid may counter the effects of L-dopa.

Calcium: Oral contraceptives and estrogen-replacement therapy may increase calcium absorption. Calcium decreases the effects of oral tetracycline.

Chromium: Chromium may reduce blood sugar levels and, in diabetics, decrease insulin requirements.

Iron: Milk, coffee, tea, and vitamin E decrease iron absorption.

Magnesium: Diuretic drugs increase requirements for magnesium. Magnesium decreases the effect of digitalis. Do not use when kidney disease is manifest. Magnesium overdose will result in diarrhea.

Selenium: Extremely high doses of selenium may cause dizziness, cardiomyopathy, and paralysis.

Zinc: Diuretic drugs increase zinc requirements.

VITAMIN-MINERAL SYNERGISMS*

Vitamin	Synergistic Minerals
A	zinc, potassium, phosphorus, magnesium, manganese, selenium
B1	selenium, cobalt, sodium, potassium, iron, manganese, magnesium, copper, zinc, phosphorus
B2	iron, phosphorus, magnesium, zinc, potassium, chromium
B3	zinc, potassium, iron, phosphorus, magnesium, sodium, chromium, selenium
B6	zinc, chromium, magnesium, sodium, potassium, phosphorus, iron, manganese, selenium
B12	selenium, copper, calcium, cobalt, sodium
pantothenic acid	chromium, sodium, potassium, zinc, phosphorus
C	iron, copper, calcium, cobalt, sodium
D	calcium, magnesium, sodium, copper, selenium
E	sodium, potassium, calcium, iron, manganese, zinc, phosphorus, selenium

*SYNERGISM: The joint action of agents, such as nutrients, that increase each other's effectiveness when taken together.
Source: Dr. David L. Watts

VITAMIN SYNERGISMS

Vitamin	Synergistic Vitamins
A	B2, C, E, B3, B1, B6
B1	E, C, B6, B12, B3, pantothenic acid, A, folic acid, B2
B2	A, B3, folic acid
B3	B1, B2, B6, A, pantothenic acid, E, folic acid
B6	E, A, B1, B3, pantothenic acid, B12, folic acid
B12	B1, B3, B6, E, pantothenic acid, C, folic acid, D
pantothenic acid	C, E, A, B1, B3, B6, folic acid
C	A, E, B6, B3, pantothenic acid
D	B12, E
E	A, B6, C, B12, B1, pantothenic acid, B3, folic acid, D

Source: Dr. David L. Watts

MINERAL SYNERGISMS

Mineral	Synergistic Minerals
calcium	magnesium, phosphorus, copper, sodium, potassium, selenium
copper	iron, cobalt, calcium, sodium, selenium
chromium	magnesium, zinc, potassium
iron	copper, manganese, potassium, sodium, chromium, phosphorus, selenium
magnesium	calcium, potassium, zinc, manganese, phosphorus, chromium
manganese	potassium, zinc, magnesium, iron, phosphorus
phosphorus	calcium, magnesium, sodium, potassium, zinc, iron
potassium	sodium, magnesium, manganese, zinc, phosphorus, iron
selenium	sodium, potassium, copper, manganese, iron, calcium
sodium	potassium, selenium, cobalt, calcium, iron, copper, phosphorus
zinc	potassium, magnesium, manganese, chromium, phosphorus

People with these sympathetic diseases:

anxiety

Source: Dr. David L. Watts

rheumatoid arthritis
histamine allergies
amyotropic lateral sclerosis (ALS)
hypertension
hyperthyroidism
hyperadrenia
Hodgkin's disease
leukemia
bacterial infections
myasthenia gravis
multiple sclerosis
peptic or duodenal ulcers
juvenile-onset diabetes

may need these sedative nutrients:
Minerals: calcium, magnesium, zinc, copper, chromium
Vitamins: D, B2, B12, choline

People with these parasympathetic diseases:

osteoarthritis
low-histamine allergies
asthma
AIDS
anorexia
fungus
hypotension
hypothyroidism
hypoadrenia
viral infections
lupus
premenstrual syndrome
Candida albicans
gastric ulcers
adult-onset (type II) diabetes

may need these stimulatory nutrients:
Minerals: phosphorus, sodium, potassium, iron, manganese, selenium
Vitamins: A, C, E, B1, B6, folic acid

Source: Dr. David L. Watts

Applying Your Nutritional Knowledge in Prevention and Treatment

How do you put your knowledge of vitamins and minerals into practice? Before you start taking vitamins or minerals, or changing the ones you're already taking, consider whether you want to follow a *moderate*, a *mildly aggressive*, or a *very aggressive* vitamin-mineral program.

Moderate Program: Are you taking, or do you want to start taking, supplements simply as a nutritional insurance policy? If your answer is yes, begin by taking a high-potency multi-vitamin and multi-mineral supplement, and consider taking extra vitamins C and E and magnesium.

Be prepared, however, to move to a mildly aggressive program as you get older. That's because the vitamins you took between the ages of 20 to 30 will be used less efficiently by your cells as you age. You will probably have to increase your supplements overall between the ages of 30 and 50. And past 50, when your risk of degenerative diseases increases sharply, you may have to increase your vitamin intake even further.

Mildly Aggressive Program: Are you taking supplements to reduce a known disease risk, such as a family history of high blood pressure, cancer, multiple sclerosis, or diabetes—even though you have no overt symptoms? In these instances, you may want to follow a mildly aggressive vitamin program.

To do so, establish a baseline supplemental intake with a multi-vitamin and multi-mineral supplement. Next, *gradually* add larger amounts of single nutrients. For example, you might consider taking 500 mg of vitamin C daily, increasing to 3 to 4 grams over 12 months. Pay attention to how your body feels: are you getting fewer colds, are your colds less severe, do you have some relief from allergies? Similarly, try taking 100 IU of vitamin E daily, increasing to 400 IU over the course of a year.

Very Aggressive Program: Are you taking supplements to treat specific diseases that you have? If this is the case, work with your physician—or, at the very least, let him know what you're doing. Odds are that you're already taking some medication if you're suffering from cancer or a type of heart disease (high blood pressure, arrhythmias, angina pectoris), diabetes, multiple sclerosis, or Parkinson's disease. It may be dangerous to simply stop taking your medicine. By working with your doctor, the two of you can titrate, or adjust, your medication and your vitamins and minerals so they work together. For example, calcium supplements are an effective treatment of high blood pressure. However, simply ceasing a prescription blood pressure medication may result in a dangerous rebound, even if you take calcium.

If your doctor has been keeping up with the latest findings on nutritional therapies, he'll probably cooperate. If he's nutritionally naïve, he may say that the vitamins or minerals you're taking (or want to take) won't help. If that's his response, show him this book and urge him to check the references at his medical library. If he's still reluctant, consider finding another doctor—remember, he's supposed to be working *for you*, not the other way around. In the meantime, you may have to decide how much of your medical treatment you want to take into your own hands.

Finally, remember that vitamins and minerals—as good as they are—are not magic bullets. For example, water is essential, but if you were to consume only water and nothing else, you would eventually die. Likewise, you shouldn't depend on a single vitamin supplement—or on vitamin supplements alone. To improve your health, consider the state of your overall diet and whether you should reduce your consumption of sugar and other highly refined foods. In addition, weigh the health benefits of still other types of nutritional supplements, such as amino acids, omega-3 fatty acids, and herbs. If feeling good always seems just beyond your grasp, consider whether you might be suffering from food and/or chemical allergies. While vitamin C will reduce an allergic response, it is best to simply avoid a food or chemical allergen whenever possible.

Vitamins, Linus Pauling has noted, are extremely powerful substances. A lack of them can lead to death, and a mediocre intake can leave you in "ordinary poor health." Taking optimal amounts of vitamins and minerals can promote the many natural and necessary biochemical processes that fight disease and maintain health. Ultimately, you—and not your doctor—must make the most of them.

Do You Have a Right to Treat Yourself?

The evidence supporting the role of vitamins and minerals in preventing—and, particularly, treating—disease is compelling. What you've read here is only the tip of the proverbial iceberg. A scan of

Medline or other medical computer databases reveals that thousands of supportive articles on vitamins and minerals are published each year.

But even with strong scientific support, do we have a "right" to treat ourselves instead of always relying on physicians? Although the right to take vitamins isn't explicitly guaranteed by the Constitution, I believe you do have an inalienable right to treat yourself. In fact, there is ample historical precedent for self-therapy. For thousands of years, and in every society and culture, people have treated themselves with herbs. As a testament to the value of herbs, 38 percent of all drugs on the market are derived from plants or synthesized based on plant chemistry.[89] Even the "wonder drug" taxol, used in treating ovarian cancer, was until 1993 extracted from the bark of the Pacific yew tree.

People continue to treat themselves every day—and, unfortunately, with substances far more dangerous than herbs and vitamins. They take aspirin. They take cough medicine. They take antihistamines—even when their value is questionable. Look at the thousands of products on the shelf of any drug store, and it's evident that people don't just have a right to treat themselves. They're *urged* to treat themselves.

So what's wrong with taking vitamins? Despite what you might hear from critics, there's absolutely nothing wrong with self-therapy with vitamins and minerals. Using them to prevent disease or treat disease is justified scientifically. Any doctor who tells you otherwise has failed to keep up with what's being published in the medical literature. Just insist that he or she check any medical database, and he'll find more proof than he has time to read. Remember, taking vitamin supplements is your right. Don't ever let anyone deny that right or take it away from you out of ignorance.

REFERENCES

1. Williams, R. J., *Biochemical Individuality: the Basis for the Genotrophic Concept*, Wiley, 1956.
2. Williams, R. J., *Nutrition Against Disease*, Pitman, 1971.
3. Williams, R. J., *Executive Health* newsletter, May 1976.
4. Challem, J. J., *Bestways*, October 1977.
5. Ibid.
6. Telephone interview with Dr. Jeffrey Blumberg, September 28, 1992.
7. Telephone interview with Dr. Emanuel Cheraskin, October 26, 1992.
8. Wallace, D. C., *Science*, May 1, 1992; 256:628–32.
9. Pauling, L., *Science*, April 1968; 160:265–71.
10. Telephone interview with Dr. Linus Pauling, October 26, 1992.
11. Stone, I., *The Healing Factor: Vitamin C Against Disease*, Grosset & Dunlap, 1972.
12. Challem, J. J., *Vitamin C Updated*, Keats Publishing, 1983.
13. Stone, I., *The Healing Factor: Vitamin C Against Disease*, Grosset & Dunlap, 1972.
14. Garewal, H., *Journal of Nutrition*, March 1992; 122(3 Suppl):728–32.
15. Coodley, G., *Journal of Acquired Immune Deficiency Syndrome*, March 1993; 6:272-6.
16. Telephone interview with Dr. Gregg Coodley, February 4, 1993.
17. Garewal, H., paper presented at the meeting of the American Society of Clinical Oncology, San Francisco, 1989.
18. Garewal, H. *American Journal of Clinical Nutrition*, January 1991; 53(1 Suppl):294S–297S.
19. *Berkeley Wellness Letter*, Feb. 13, 1990.
20. *Cancer Weekly*, Nov. 13, 1989.
21. Stampfer, M., *JAMA*, Aug. 19, 1989; 268:877–81.
22. Manore, M., *American Journal of Clinical Nutrition*, Aug. 1989; 50:339–45.

23. Subar, A., *American Journal of Clinical Nutrition*, Sept. 1989; 50:508–16.
24. Clarke, R., *New England Journal of Medicine*, April 25, 1991; 324:1149–55.
25. Israelsson, B., *Atherosclerosis*, June 1988; 71:227–33.
26. Ellis, J., *Annals of the New York Academy of Sciences*. 1990; 585:295–301.
27. Reynolds, E., *Archives of Neurology*, August 1991; 48:808–811.
28. Reynolds, E., *Archives of Neurology*, June 1992; 49:649–52.
29. Braunwald E., (editor), *Heart Disease: A Textbook of Cardiovascular Medicine*, 3rd edition, W. B. Saunders Co., 1988, page 1169.
30. Kane, J., *Journal of the American Medical Association*, Dec. 19, 1990; 264:3007–12.
31. *Newsweek*, May 18, 1992.
32. *The Oregonian*, May 8, 1992.
33. Enstrom, J., *Epidemiology*, May 1992; Vol. 3:194–202.
34. Hemilä, H., *British Journal of Medicine*, 67:3–16.
35. Pauling, L. and E. Cameron, *Cancer and Vitamin C*, The Linus Pauling Institute of Science and Medicine, 1979.
36. Interview with Dr. Linus Pauling, May 1990, Vancouver, Canada.
37. Telephone interview with Dr. Linus Pauling, Oct. 22, 1992.
38. Ibid.
39. Rath, M. and L. Pauling, *Journal of Orthomolecular Medicine*, 1992; 7:5–15.
40. Hemilä, H., *Journal of Hypertension*, 1991; 9:1076–1078.
41. Verlangieri, A., *Life Sciences*, 1990; 46:619–24.
42. Salonen, J., *Circulation*, Sept. 1992; 86:803–811.
43. There is some dispute as to whether all forms of iron supplements or just the inorganic forms of iron supplements are antagonistic with vitamin E. It's easy enough to take one supplement in the morning and the other in the evening to minimize the problem.
44. Riemersma, R., *Vitamin E: Biochemistry and Health Implications*, *Annals of the New York Academy of Sciences*, 1989; 570:291–5.
45. Riemersma, R., *Lancet*, Jan. 5, 1991; 337:1–5.
46. Verlangieri, A., *Journal of the American College of Nutrition*, April 1992; 11:131–8.
47. Jialal, I., *Journal of Lipid Research*, June 1992; 3:899–906.
48. Jandak, J., *Blood*, 1989; 73:141–9.
49. Jandak, J., *Thrombosis Research*, 1988; 49:393–404.
50. Gridley, G., *American Journal of Epidemiology*, June 15, 1992, 135:1083–1092.
51. *Journal of the National Cancer Institute*, July 1, 1992; 84:996–7.
52. Knekt, P., *American Journal of Epidemiology*, 1988; 127:28–41.

53. Knekt, P., *International Journal of Epidemiology*, 1988; 17:281–88.
54. Sokol, R., *Annual Review of Nutrition*, 1988; 8:351–73.
55. LeBel, P., *Biochemical and Biophysical Research Communications*, September 15, 1989; 163:860–6.
56. Cadet, J. L., *Vitamin E: Biochemistry and Health Implications, Annals of the New York Academy of Sciences*, 1989; 570:176–185.
57. Fahn, S., *Annals of the New York Academy of Sciences*, 1989; 570:186–96.
58. Golbe, L., *Archives of Neurology*, 1988; 45:1350–3.
59. *Science News*, Nov. 21, 1992; 142:340.
60. McCarron, D., *Science*, June 29, 1984; 224:1392–98.
61. Sato, K., *Hypertension*, March 1989; 13:219–226.
62. Belizan, J., *New England Journal of Medicine*, Nov. 14, 1991; 325:1399–1405.
63. McGarvey, S., *Hypertension*, Feb. 1991; 17:218–24.
64. McCarron, D., *American Journal of Clinical Nutrition*, July 1991; 54:215S–19S.
65. McCarron, D., *Hypertension*, Jan. 1991; 17(suppl I):I-170–I-172.
66. Kanis, J. A., *British Medical Journal*, 1989; 298:205–8.
67. Reid, I., *New England Journal of Medicine*, Feb. 18, 1993; 328:460–4.
68. Heaney, R., *New England Journal of Medicine*, Feb. 18, 1993; 328:503–5.
69. Nordin, C., *British Medical Journal*, 1990; 300:1056–60.
70. Nelson, M., *American Journal of Clinical Nutrition*, May 1991; 53:1304–11.
71. Woods, K., *Lancet*, June 27, 1992; 339:1553–58.
72. Smith, L., *International Journal of Cardiology*, 1986; 12:175–80.
73. Ceremuzynski, L., *American Heart Journal*, Dec. 1989; 118:1333–4.
74. Keren, A., *PACE*, July 1990; 13:937–45.
75. *Science News*, Sept. 22, 1990.
76. Mooradian, A. *American Journal of Clinical Nutrition*, 1987; 45:877–95.
77. Altura, B., *Proceedings of the National Academy of Sciences*, March 1990; 87:1840–44.
78. Singh, R., *Magnesium*, Sept.–Oct. 1990; 9:255–64.
79. Evans, G., *Western Journal of Medicine*, Jan. 1990; 152:41–45.
80. Ji, L., *Journal of the American College of Nutrition*, Feb. 1992; 11:79–86.
81. Birt, D., *Magnesium*, Jan.–Feb. 1989; 8:17–30.
82. Knekt, P., *International Journal of Epidemiology*, 1988; 17:281–88.
83. Knekt, P., *International Journal of Cancer*, 1988; 42:846–50.
84. Halcomb, W. *Antimicrobial Agents and Chemotherapy*, 1984; 25:20–24.
85. Godfrey, J., *Journal of International Medical Research*, 1992; 20:234–46.

85. Godfrey, J., *Journal of International Medical Research*, 1992; 20:234–46.

86. *Science News*, May 4, 1991.

87. Watts, D., *Journal of Orthomolecular Medicine*, 1990; 5:11–19.

88. For more information on vitamin-mineral-drug interactions, see Griffith, H., *The Complete Guide to Vitamins, Minerals & Supplements*, 1988, Fisher Books, Tucson, AZ.

89. Morton, I., *Major Medicinal Plants: Botany, Culture and Uses*, Charles C. Thomas Publisher, 1977.

Good Health Guides for Areas of Special Interest